G000124252

1,000,000 Books

are available to read at

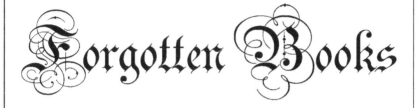

---

www.ForgottenBooks.com

Read online
Download PDF
Purchase in print

ISBN 978-1-397-32530-3
PIBN 11374493

This book is a reproduction of an important historical work. Forgotten Books uses
state-of-the-art technology to digitally reconstruct the work, preserving the original format
whilst repairing imperfections present in the aged copy. In rare cases, an imperfection in
the original, such as a blemish or missing page, may be replicated in our edition. We do,
however, repair the vast majority of imperfections successfully; any imperfections that
remain are intentionally left to preserve the state of such historical works.

Forgotten Books is a registered trademark of FB &c Ltd.
Copyright © 2018 FB &c Ltd.
FB &c Ltd, Dalton House, 60 Windsor Avenue, London, SW19 2RR.
Company number 08720141. Registered in England and Wales.

For support please visit www.forgottenbooks.com

1 MONTH OF
FREE
READING

at

www.ForgottenBooks.com

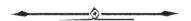

By purchasing this book you are eligible for one month membership to ForgottenBooks.com, giving you unlimited access to our entire collection of over 1,000,000 titles via our web site and mobile apps.

To claim your free month visit:

www.forgottenbooks.com/free1374493

* Offer is valid for 45 days from date of purchase. Terms and conditions apply.

English
Français
Deutsche
Italiano
Español
Português

www.forgottenbooks.com

Mythology Photography **Fiction**
Fishing Christianity **Art** Cooking
Essays Buddhism Freemasonry
Medicine **Biology** Music **Ancient
Egypt** Evolution Carpentry Physics
Dance Geology **Mathematics** Fitness
Shakespeare **Folklore** Yoga Marketing
Confidence Immortality Biographies
Poetry **Psychology** Witchcraft
Electronics Chemistry History **Law**
Accounting **Philosophy** Anthropology
Alchemy Drama Quantum Mechanics
Atheism Sexual Health **Ancient History**
Entrepreneurship Languages Sport
Paleontology Needlework Islam
Metaphysics Investment Archaeology
Parenting Statistics Criminology
Motivational

U.S. WAR DEPARTMENT

PAMPHLET No. 8-3

HEALTH PRECAUTIONS
FOR
AFRICAN AND ASIATIC COUNTRIES ALONG SOUTHERN AND EASTERN MEDITERRANEAN SEA, RED SEA, AND PERSIAN GULF

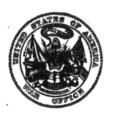

1943

UNITED STATES
GOVERNMENT PRINTING OFFICE
WASHINGTON : 1943

QT
150
U63h
1943
c. 1

No part of this pamphlet may be published without the permission of
The Surgeon General, United States Army

WAR DEPARTMENT,
WASHINGTON, April 20, 1943.

HEALTH PRECAUTIONS FOR AFRICAN AND ASIATIC COUNTRIES ALONG SOUTHERN AND EASTERN MEDITERRANEAN SEA, RED SEA, AND PERSIAN GULF

1. **General.**—*a.* Military personnel and other travelers in Northern and Eastern Africa and the Western Asiatic countries are exposed to serious health hazards, both because of the presence of diseases not commonly encountered in the United States and the relatively high incidence of certain other diseases that normally occur in North America. Some of the countries included in this general area have acceptable health departments, and a few of the larger cities have good health organizations, especially those under British influence. In normal times these health organizations may compare with those of some of the cities of the United States. However, viewed as a whole, and considering the influence of the war, health conditions are much less satisfactory than in our country, and the traveler who values his health must be alert at all times to the possibility of illness and must guard against it by observing certain necessary hygienic and sanitary precautions. Carelessness in this respect may result in the acquisition of diseases, some of which may be serious, but proper application of known health precautions should obviate all or most disability for persons temporarily assigned to live in this part of the world.

b. This pamphlet is designed to cover the potential hazards of a large general area, so that all the conditions enumerated may not apply to a limited locality. Common sense and good judgment, together with information acquired from local health authorities and Army medical officers, should serve to indicate which of the precautions outlined below can be modified or dispensed with to meet local conditions. These brief statements are not intended as a substitute for the broad preventive medicine program of the Army.

2. Water.—*a.* Drinking water contaminated with human fecal matter is one of the most common sources of infections of the intestinal tract, including the common diarrheas, typhoid fever, the paratyphoid fevers, amebic dysentery, bacillary dysentery, and, in some areas, cholera, and schistosomiasis. Dracontiasis (Guinea worm infection) may also be acquired from water. Improper methods of disposal of human wastes and inadequate treatment of water contaminated by these wastes are direct causes of impure water. Facilities for the treatment of water usually are found only in cities and in oil company settlements located at fields and at stations along the pipe lines. However, even in cities the water frequently is not safe because of inadequate equipment, lack of supervision of water purification facilities, or both. In certain instances, safe water is produced at the water plant, but it is contaminated while passing through faulty water mains or by being carried in insanitary containers (tins, jars, animal skins, etc.). In many cities, water distribution systems reach only a limited area and thus supply only a small percentage of the inhabitants, usually those in the European settlements.

b. The probability of outbreaks of various communicable diseases, especially water- and food-borne diseases, is greatly increased as a result of religious pilgrimages to Mecca and other shrines from all parts of the Mohammedan world.

c. While safe water may be found in some localities in Moslem countries of Northern Africa and Western Asia, for the health protection of Army personnel traveling widely in this part of the world it is generally advisable to consider all water as unsafe for human consumption. Ice frozen from these waters presents the same problem as the water itself, and is unsafe for use in drinks.

d. Carbonated drinks made from local water supplies should not be regarded as altogether safe. Soft drinks (noncarbonated, for example, orangeade, etc.) are dangerous unless known to be prepared under hygienic conditions and pasteurized. They should not be consumed unless the source is known to be reliable.

e. Liquids recommended as safe for human consumption are—

    (1) Boiled water (boiled from 3 to 5 minutes).

(2) Water properly treated with chlorine (see below; see also par. 20c(4) and (5), FM 21–10, as changed by C 4, January 16, 1943).

(3) Tea ⎫
(4) Coffee ⎬ When water is boiled in preparation of these drinks.

(5) Beer and wines, when properly prepared and bottled.

(6) Fruit juices, undiluted, and freshly prepared by oneself.

(7) Water treated under the supervision of British or United States Army Medical Department personnel is safe and should be used where available.

f. Proper chlorination of water requires care and attention to details, regardless of the amount treated. If large quantities are to be purified, the Lyster bag may be used as described in paragraph 20c, FM 21–10. For individual use, either halazone tablets or calcium hypochlorite powder may be used in canteens.

g. If halazone is used, two tablets (4.0 mg. or $\frac{1}{16}$ grain each) are required for each canteen (1 quart) of water. If the water is especially turbid, one or two additional tablets may be necessary. Where high-test calcium hypochlorite is used, the procedure is as follows: The standard Army tube is broken and the contents dissolved in a canteen of water. One canteen-top full (approximately 1½ teaspoons) of this mixture may then be added to each full canteen of water which is to be treated. Regardless of the method used, the water should be allowed to stand for ½ hour, after which the "odor" or "taste" test should be applied. If the odor of free chlorine can be detected or chlorine tasted when the water is applied to the tongue, a chlorine content of at least 0.4 parts per million is indicated, and the water may be considered safe. Be certain that the odor of chlorine does not come from concentrated chlorine spilled on the hands or the water container by careless handling. When practicable, some form of filtration should be employed if the water is turbid or contains large amounts of organic material. This will also aid in eliminating the encysted form of the organism which causes amebic dysentery.

h. Water used for washing the teeth or washing toothbrushes requires the same treatment as drinking water.

i. Liquids should be taken only from glasses or other containers that are known to be clean.

3. Water economy under desert conditions.—*a.* Day temperatures may go as high as 130° F. in desert climates, which subjects the human body to severe physiological stress, especially regarding loss of water and salt. Exertion under these conditions is accompanied by copious sweating. As a result of such sweating not only are large quantities of fluid (water) lost, but also much body salt which is in solution in the sweat. Under extreme conditions, as much as 10 quarts of water daily may be lost by perspiration, although in hot dry climates so much evaporation occurs that one is not conscious of increased sweating. In fact, evaporation of sweat in high temperatures is the principal method by which the body is able to cool itself and thus maintain a normal temperature.

b. In temperate climates, except under conditions of strenuous physical exertion during warm weather, salt and water lost by excretion are replaced by a normal diet and a moderate fluid intake; however, in the heat of the desert, excess salt and fluids must be ingested in order to maintain normal body requirements for these chemicals. Experience of desert armies indicates that an average of about 1½ gallons of water per man per day may be all that can be supplied for all personal purposes. Under extremes of temperature and physical exertion, up to 3 gallons are likely to be necessary. In emergencies, ¾ gallon per day may suffice, but on such a restricted water intake physical efficiency is reduced after a short interval, probably 2 or 3 days. Therefore, under desert conditions where water supplies are inadequate, *it is imperative to conserve water* both before consumption by care of water supplies and after ingestion by *limiting to a minimum* physical exertion and exposure to the sun, thus reducing unnecessary sweating. Salt lost in perspiration should be replaced (see *c*(3) below).

c. Precautions.

(1) Stay in the shade, *out of the sun,* as much as possible. Heavy work should be done at night, very early in the morning, or late in the afternoon. When work during the hot hours of the day is mandatory, frequent periods of rest are necessary.

(2) Drink water slowly and in small amounts (not more than 6 to 8 ounces at a time), but more frequently than in temperate climates.

(3) Take two tablets of salt (equivalent to 20 grains, 1.3 grams, or ¼ teaspoonful) with every canteen of water (1 quart) consumed. See Circular No. 129, War Department, 1941, and Circular No. 169, War Department, 1941.

(4) Avoid unnecessary physical exertion, and thereby prevent excessive perspiration.

(5) Wear headgear, preferably a sun helmet, when exposure to the sun is necessary for an appreciable period of time. Outer garments should be loose-fitting to facilitate evaporation of perspiration. Shorts may be worn with benefit during the day, especially indoors, but from dusk

until morning long trousers and long sleeves are imperative. The often-repeated suggestions to wear abdominal
bands, spinal pads, and such contrivances to prevent
diarrheas have no scientific basis and are detrimental
since they interfere with normal heat loss from the body.

(6) Cool water evaporates more slowly and is more palatable
than warm water. Protect water supplies by keeping
them in closed containers in the shade. Use insulated
containers where possible.

(7) Where conditions permit, such foods as canned tomatoes
may be advantageous not only as rations, but also because they supply additional fluids.

(8) Fluids are lost not only by excess perspiration, but also
through vomiting and diarrhea. Individuals suffering
from these conditions, or from illnesses accompanied by
fever, are susceptible to the effects of heat and should
not be sent out from bases or camps until recovery has
been complete.

4. **Foods.**—*a. General.*

(1) Foods are the second great source of the intestinal diseases.
They assume even greater hazards for the uninitiated or
unwary, due to the fact that not only are foods subject
to contamination as in the case of water, but also because
they are culture media for the growth of bacteria. Refrigeration facilities for preventing or reducing bacterial
growth (spoilage) in foods, especially meats and milk,
are inadequate or lacking in many localities in this part of
the world. In most instances meat is not inspected, either
before or after slaughter, so that meat from animals infected with tuberculosis, undulant fever, anthrax, trichi-
nosis, etc., may be distributed for human consumption.
Heat (cooking) is the only practical and effective agent
for destroying bacteria in foods, but even well-cooked
foods are subject to recontamination by food handlers
(cooks and waiters) or by flies and other insects and
small animals, and thus may become unsafe for consumption. Only well-cooked foods, freshly prepared, preferably consumed while hot, and not reheated, are safe for
human consumption. Exceptions are bread and crackers,
which may be considered safe unless mechanically
contaminated.

(2) Foods for lunches, as commonly prepared before short
missions (flights, patrols, etc.) in the United States, are

likely to spoil in a short time under tropical or desert conditions. Therefore, it is recommended that sandwiches should not be made before departure, but that such foods as canned meats and other tinned goods, bread, crackers, thick-skinned fruits, etc., be carried. The Army tinned field ration is a practical safe food for the above uses. If canned foods are used, they must be eaten soon after the can is opened.

b. *Milk.*

(1) Improperly handled dairy products (milk, cream, butter, etc.) constitute one of the most dangerous groups of foods. Inspected disease-free dairy herds, pasteurization, and adequate refrigeration are not commonly encountered in Asia or Northern Africa. Raw milk not subjected to these safeguards may carry the following diseases: dysentery, typhoid and paratyphoid fevers, common diarrheas, diphtheria, tuberculosis, undulant fever, septic sore throat, and other infectious diseases.

(2) Only properly bottled pasteurized milk (meeting Medical Department standards), canned evaported milk, condensed milk, powdered milk prepared with boiled water, or milk boiled immediately before use can be recommended. All other milk should be considered unsafe. This also includes ice cream prepared with local milk, and cream for coffee, cereals, etc.

c. *Fruits and vegetables.*—Soil pollution by human excreta is common in this part of the world. As a result of fertilizing with human excreta, vegetables grown by the native farmers are almost certain to be contaminated. Any of the intestinal diseases may be acquired by the consumption of uncooked vegetables. The risk of amebic dysentery is especially great, since the encysted form of the ameba as passed in the stool is resistant to soap and water and is destroyed with difficulty except by heat (cooking). Therefore, only *freshly cooked* vegetables should be eaten. Such standard items of the American diet as salads made of lettuce, other uncooked leafy vegetables, raw carrots, and other root vegetables cannot be eaten with safety. The dipping of vegetables in chemical solutions such as potassium permanganate *does not* protect against intestinal infections. Thick-skinned fruits requiring peeling, for example, citrus fruits, papayas, mangoes, and melons, are safe for human consumption provided they are not mixed with raw vegetables in salads. It is considered advisable to scald the skins of these fruits before peeling and eating.

5. Clothing.—*a.* The prevalence of certain skin diseases, partienlarly "dhobie itch," necessitates frequent change of underclothing and socks. Lightweight clothing suitable for summer wear in the southern United States is satisfactory except in certain mountainous areas and in Iraq and Iran, where winter temperatures as low as 0° F. may be anticipated (January). Marked variations of temperature between day and night in the desert necessitate both warm and tropical types of clothing. Cases of pneumonia have been reported in increased numbers among aviators flying under desert conditions, and are thought to be due, in part, to the drastic change from the high temperature of ground levels to the cold of altitude, and vice versa, without an opportunity to change to suitable clothing for either one extreme or the other.

b. Care should be taken to put on a sweat shirt, jacket, or similar garment immediately after violent exertion. Suitable headgear, preferably a sun helmet, is required when exposure to the sun is necessary. Shoes should be worn at all times as a precaution against hookworm disease. Because of the prevalence of certain eye diseases, for example, trachoma, gonorrheal ophthalmitis, and Koch-Weeks ophthalmia (pink eye), it is necessary to avoid contact with towels, pillowcases, bed clothing, and similar personal articles used by other individuals.

6. Bathing; swimming.—*a.* Daily bathing is essential where the water supply will permit. It is important to clean and dry thoroughly all skin folds of the body (between the toes, crotch, groin, around the scrotum, and the armpits) in order to prevent fungus infections such as "dhobie itch." The use of Army-issue foot powder daily on the parts of the body noted above is also a good preventive measure. If skin rashes or infections appear, a medical officer should be consulted as soon as practicable.

b. Fresh waters, such as lakes, rivers, streams, swamps, irrigation ditches, flooded rice fields, etc., in the area covered by this survey often harbor the young forms (larvae) of various blood worms or flukes. These flukes enter the body through the skin of swimmers or bathers or persons wading in such waters and may cause serious diseases of the bladder and intestines. The diseases noted above are known as urinary bilharziasis or schistosomiasis and intestinal bilharziasis or schistosomiasis, respectively. An early symptom of these diseases may be a skin rash. The urinary type is more common in this part of the world and in some areas affects from 20 to 40 percent of the native population. It is also possible to become infected with these flukes by drinking contaminated water that has not been boiled or sufficiently treated with chlorine. The larvae are harbored by several species of fresh-water snails, and when discharged into the water cannot survive longer than 48 to 72 hours without another suitable host. Thus, if water for bathing is stored in a clean container for such a time, and is free of snails, it becomes safe for bathing purposes. This does not insure water satisfactory for drinking. Since the larvae do not live in sea water, salt-water bathing and swimming, except at beaches near the mouths of fresh-water streams or near city sewage outlets, present no disease hazard.

7. **Housing.**—Native homes and dwellings are often filthy, harboring insects and pests of many descriptions. Walls and furnishings of tents and dwellings, especially rugs and floor mats that are used as beds, usually are infested with lice, fleas, bedbugs, and/or other insects. It is wise to refrain from sleeping in these places. Dangerous and obnoxious vermin, such as snakes and scorpions, are common in this area, and many species prefer to live in close proximity to man. They may enter houses and crawl into such warm dark places as shoes, clothing, luggage, and bureau drawers; consequently these articles should be inspected carefully before use. Avoid dogs and other small animals kept as household pets in many dwellings, since they may be carriers of rabies as well as harborers of ticks and fleas. Native habitations should be avoided as much as possible. Every effort should be made to secure clean and tightly screened quarters. Each individual should carry his own mosquito net.

8. **Insect carriers of disease.**—There are numerous species of insects of importance to man, many only of a pestilential nature, others important as vectors of serious diseases. The most important insect carriers of disease are listed below, with brief discussions of the diseases that they may carry and the applicable precautionary measures.

　a. Mosquitoes.

　　(1) *Malaria.*

　　　　(*a*) Malaria, spread only by the bite of female anopheline mosquitoes, is a serious disease, the danger of which in many parts of Asia and Africa cannot be overestimated. It is unusually prevalent along the coasts of the Mediterranean Sea, the Red Sea, and the Persian Gulf, and follows the river courses inland. Malarial mosquitoes are also to be found in the oases, along irrigation canals and ditches, and some varieties have adapted themselves to desert conditions and are able to breed in mere trickles of water. Others breed in caves, wells, cisterns, or cesspools. Certain varieties of malaria-carrying mosquitoes are also found in the mountains, where they may tolerate altitudes of 6,000 to 8,000 feet. Malaria is unusually prevalent in the hills and mountains of northeastern Iraq and in the mountains of Iran.

(b) These mosquitoes feed during dusk or at night and occasionally during the day where the light is greatly reduced, as in deep-shaded jungles. Along the seacoasts, rivers, and marshy subcoastal areas in some countries (notably Egypt, Iraq, Iran, and Palestine) great numbers of mosquitoes are found and malaria is prevalent.

(c) Man is the reservoir of malaria. Up to 80 percent or more of the native inhabitants of some regions are infected with this disease. Anopheline mosquitoes become infected when they feed on (bite) a human being who has malaria. After an incubation period of from 14 to 40 days these mosquitoes are capable of transmitting the disease.

(d) Several varieties of malaria-carrying mosquitoes breed in small collections of water about houses and, unless care is taken, may enter buildings through carelessly opened screen doors, torn screens, cracks, spaces formed by the junction of corrugated or tiled roofs and walls, etc. During the day these mosquitoes hide in corners and other parts of the house where there is little light, but come out to feed after dark.

(e) *Preventive measures.*

1. Sleep in screened rooms or under mosquito nets. Inspect screens, doors, and mosquito nets at regular intervals, and search for live mosquitoes in those parts of the house where there is little light.

2. After dark, stay indoors in properly screened buildings as much as possible.

3. When it is necessary to be out of doors after dark, move about continually.

4. If possible, select camp sites on high, windswept ground away from areas infested with mosquitoes, and *far removed from native villages* (the inhabitants of which are often infected and act as a reservoir of malaria).

(f) *Additional measures that may be applicable.*

    1. The use of head nets, gloves, and mosquito boots, along with other mosquitoproof clothing covering the entire body. (Mosquitoes are able to bite through the material ordinarily used in shirts and other lightweight clothing.)

    2. Mosquito repellants applied to all exposed parts of the body at regular intervals.

    3. Insecticide sprays used inside airplanes and in living quarters in the early morning and late afternoon, and at other times when necessary.

    4. The use of quinine or atabrine for suppressive treatment (prophylaxis) is not recommended as a routine procedure, since the available information indicates that these drugs do not prevent infection. They are, however, of definite military value in that they do prevent clinical symptoms of malaria so long as they are taken, and thus afford a means of keeping troops fit during periods of emergency in the field. Such drugs should be used only under special conditions and when advised by medical officers, flight surgeons, or local health authorities. The present War Department policy advocates atabrine 0.1 gram (1½ grains or one tablet) twice daily after meals, on 2 days a week, allowing a 2- or 3-day interval between days of taking. If atabrine is not available, take quinine sulfate 0.64 gram (10 grains or two tablets) after the evening meal each day. (Circular Letter No. 135, dated October 21, 1942.)

    5. The estivo-autumnal type of malaria may give rise to bizarre symptoms, entirely different from the usual chills and fever. It is therefore advisable, when residing in or traveling from malarious areas, to suspect malaria when the cause of an illness is unknown, regardless of whether there is fever or not. A physician should be consulted and advised of the possibility of recent exposure.

(2) *Yellow fever.*

(*a*) Yellow fever occurs in West and Central Africa from 15° N. to 10° S. latitude. While actually the same disease, urban yellow fever and jungle yellow fever are differentiated, depending upon the mode of spread and the source of infection. Urban yellow fever is carried from infected humans to susceptible individuals by the *Aedes aegypti* mosquito, and while the sources of jungle yellow fever are not known definitely, it has been shown that certain jungle mosquitoes are naturally infected with the virus, probably from jungle animals.

(*b*) While yellow fever has never been reported in Asia, and no cases have been seen in Northern Africa in many years, the presence of the mosquito carrier is important since these mosquitoes could readily spread yellow fever in these areas if infected mosquitoes or a person ill of the disease were brought in by airplane or by other means. The disease occurs in many parts of Western and Central Africa, where sporadic cases and deaths were reported regularly during 1941 and 1942, and urban yellow fever appeared in epidemic form in the Anglo-Egyptian Sudan during December, 1940.

(*c*) The mosquito carrier, *Aedes aegypti*, a form of *Stegomyia*, is called a domestic mosquito because it breeds in tubs, pots, cisterns, and other collections of water in close proximity to man.

(*d*) The precautionary measures outlined in (1) (*e*) *1* and *4*, and (*f*) *1, 2,* and *3* above, under preventive measures against malaria, are also applicable for protection against mosquitoes that carry yellow fever. In addition, vaccination against yellow fever is required under the conditions outlined in paragraph 13.

(3) *Dengue fever.*—Dengue-fever or breakbone fever is apt to occur in any part of Northern Africa or Western Asia and is very common along the southern and eastern coasts of the Mediterranean Sea. This disease is carried by the "yellow fever mosquito" (*Aedes aegypti*), al-

11

though certain other mosquitoes may also act as vectors. These mosquitoes will feed· (bite) during the day, but usually not in bright sunlight. Precautionary measures against dengue fever are the same as for yellow fever except that there is no vaccination.

(4) *Filariasis.*

(a) There are several different types of filarial worms that can be introduced into man by mosquitoes. These small worms travel in the body by way of the lymphatic channels, frequently blocking them. While the disease ordinarily does not cause any serious incapacity, elephantiasis or chronic swelling of the legs and scrotum may develop, and it seems certain that sooner or later all individuals affected will suffer some ill effects.

(b) Since the disease is prevalent throughout this entire region, and chances for exposure are great, it is not likely that soldiers will remain unaffected by this disease. Methods for protection against malaria as outlined in (1) (e), *1, 2, 3,* and *4* and (f) *1, 2,* and *3* above, will also prove valuable in preventing filariasis.

b. *Body lice.*

(1) Body lice (*Pediculus humanus corporis*) are carriers of the *epidemic* form of typhus fever (not to be confused with typhoid fever, an intestinal disease) Typhus fever is common throughout Northern Africa and Western Asia and is particularly prevalent in Morocco, Algeria, Tunisia, and Egypt; it is less so in Iran and Iraq.

(2) The second important louse-carried disease in this part of the world is a form of relapsing fever. This disease is found throughout Asia and Africa, but is particularly prevalent in the area bordering the Red Sea. Lice also carry the micro-organism (*Rickettsia quintana*) that is thought to cause trench fever.

(3) Hygienic measures against louse-borne diseases are—

(a) Frequent bathing (when a satisfactory water supply is available).

(b) Frequent changes into freshly laundered and pressed clothing.

(c) Careful selection of sleeping quarters so that clean bed clothing (changed and laundered daily, if possible) is used.

(d) Avoid native habitations and close contact with louse-infected individuals. Avoid native crowds. Sleep and eat only in the best accommodations available.

(e) Use of Army-issue insecticide powder on the seams of clothing and on bedding as indicated.

(f) In the presence of mass louse infestation, the use of group delousing methods may be employed as outlined in paragraphs 57 to 66, inclusive, FM 21–10, and in additional instructions on delousing issued from time to time.

c. *Fleas.*—In addition to being annoying, rat fleas (*Xenopsylla cheopis*) are vectors (carriers) of at least two serious diseases affecting man, namely, plague and *endemic* (rat or murine) typhus fever. Fleas found on rats commonly carry these diseases. The finding of dead·rats or other rodents may indicate that these diseases, especially plague, are prevalent among local animals. Fleas leaving dying rodents and seeking new animal hosts are especially dangerous. Thus by infesting humans, they may transmit plague and murine typhus fever. Plague in humans (human plague or bubonic plague) was reported in 1942 in Egypt, Morocco, and Palestine. Human cases of flea-borne typhus (rat or murine typhus) are found throughout the inhabited areas of Northern Africa and Western Asia. Neither plague nor the murine form of typhus fever is likely to be of importance to individuals if the precautionary measures outlined above under "Lice" (b above) are followed, and rats and rat-infested buildings are avoided.

d. *Ticks.*

(1) Various species of ticks are found throughout Western Asia and Northern Africa. A form of relapsing fever is carried by some of these insects (*Ornithodorus papillipes*), while fievre boutonneuse or tick typhus is commouly carried by dog ticks (*Rhipicephalus sanguineus*).

(2) *Precautionary measures.*

(a) Measures outlined under "Lice" (b above).

(b) Avoid native habitations, especially at·night when the ticks come out of the walls.

(c) Avoid sleeping on the ground, particularly in long grass, or resting near the trunks of trees (ticks hide in grass and under the bark of trees during the day).

(d) Always examine bed for ticks before turning in.

(*e*) Examine skin and clothing for ticks at least twice daily. Remove all ticks and kill them. It is best to remove them with forceps or small pieces of cotton cloth or paper. If the insects are removed with the fingers, extreme care must be taken to avoid crushing,.since the excreta or the blood may cause infection with the various tick-borne diseases. The ticks are best killed by burning,.by crushing between two stones, or by similar methods.

(*f*) The site of the tick bite should be cleansed and treated with an antiseptic such as iodine or alcohol.

e. Flies.—Certain fly-borne diseases are of importance in Asia and Africa.

(1) *Common housefly* (*Musca domestica*).

(*a*) By purely mechanical means, flies are capable of carrying the causative organisms of the enteric diseases from filth and fecal matter to the food of man. Infectious material from the ulcers of yaws and Oriental sore (leishmaniasis) may be carried by flies in the same manner, and eye diseases may be transmitted mechanically by these insects.

(*b*) *General precautionary measures* (see par. 35, FM 21–10; also **AR** 40–205).

1. Destruction of flies, that is, swatting, trapping, poisoning, etc.

2. Elimination of fly breeding places, that is, careful and complete disposal of wastes and refuse (human excreta, manure, garbage, rotting fallen fruits, other organic matter).

3. Use of insect repellents or sprays.

4. Use of nettings and/or screens.

5. Protection of foods.

(2) *Fly boils* (*myiasis*).—The bites of certain types of flies found in Africa and Asia may cause deep-seated abscesses or boils that heal with difficulty in the absence of medical attention. In the process of biting or alighting, the flies deposit their eggs or larvae (maggots—grubs) in or on the skin, in open wounds, the nostrils, or ear canals. The eggs of some of these flies may be carried by other insects, for example, mosquitoes. The development of

the maggots in these locations is accompanied by bacterial infection and subsequent boil formation. Surgical removal of the growing fly larva is necessary for cure.

(3) Sandflies of the genus *Phlebotomus* transmit a virus disease known as pappataci fever or sandfly fever. This disease is of a mild nature and resembles dengue fever. It is prevalent over practically all of the East. Evidence indicates that sandflies also are capable of transmitting the organism causing Oriental sore, and may be responsible for the spread of kala-azar, a serious disease affecting many people in the Near East.

9. Animals; diseases acquired from animals.—Animals are not only the hosts for insect carriers of disease (par. 8, rat fleas, lice, dog ticks, etc.), but also may be directly responsible for the spread to man of diseases which these animals themselves contract. Animal-borne diseases likely to be encountered in Asia and Northern Africa are noted below.

a. Weil's disease is an infectious liver disease transmitted in food or water spoiled by the excreta of infected rats. Thus man can contract the disease either by eating or drinking contaminated food or drinks, or by swimming or wading in water contaminated with infected rat urine or feces.

b. Rabies (mad dog bite, hydrophobia) is acquired from domestic dogs and cats, wild jackals, wolves, foxes, etc. If bitten by an animal thought to be rabid, the wound should be cleansed as thoroughly as possible, any available antiseptic applied, and a physician consulted as soon as possible. If practicable, save the animal for observation and examination.

c. Hydatid disease or echinococcosis, a disease affecting the muscles, brain, and liver, is caused by small tapeworm larvae common in native dogs. It is found in all of the countries bordering the Mediterranean and Red Seas. The disease may be contracted by sheep, cattle, and pigs, but also attacks humans. Human infection is usually the result of eating with unclean hands soiled with dirt contaminated by dog feces, or by the ingestion of contaminated foods. Petting or fondling infected dogs is also a source of danger.

d. Anthrax is a disease of sheep, cattle, hogs, camels, and other animals. This disease may be acquired from handling infected meats or eating infected meats which have been inadequately cooked. Hides or wool of these animals and such personal articles as unsterilized hairbrushes or shaving brushes made from animal hair or bristles also are possible sources of anthrax.

e. Snake bite.

(1) There are several varieties of poisonous snakes found throughout this part of the world, and snake bite is not uncommon. Cobras (*Elapidae*), vipers (*Viperidae*), and pit vipers (*Crotalinae*) are indigenous, and a poisonous sea snake (*Hydrophidae*) is found from the Persian Gulf southward.

(2) In case of snake bite, it is important to kill the snake and have it examined. There are several different types of snake antivenom, and unless the snake is identified, the specific antivenom for the treatment of the bite of the particular species of snake cannot be selected. However, in many localities it is probable that the only antivenom available will be effective against all important types of venom (polyvalent). The presence of an undigested or partially digested "ball" of food in the snake's stomach may indicate the amount of venom injected into the victim when the snake bit. When a venomous snake kills, a part of its venom is used up; thus the presence of a visible food ball in its stomach may mean that its poison sacs were relatively empty and therefore that probably only a small amount of venom was injected when the snake bit.

(3) *Precautions.*

(a) Wear boots when required to walk in snake-infested areas.

(b) Avoid the careless touching of shrubs, brush, trees, tree branches, etc., or walking near ledges where snakes may be hiding.

(c) Examine clothing and shoes before getting dressed and always look in cupboards, drawers, and other dark places before reaching into them.

(d) Have a flashlight or other source of light available at the bedside, so that the floor may be examined before getting out of bed in the night.

(e) If bitten by a snake, the following procedures are recommended:

1. Immediately apply pressure or tourniquet (rubber tubing, belt, piece of shirt, string, vine, or weed) above the bite, no tighter than a snug garter, to stop the venous blood return toward the heart. The tourniquet should be released for a few seconds every 10 to 15 minutes to prevent gangrene.

2. Under field conditions and in the absence of medical care, *do not* make an incision, but instead place a 3- or 4-inch square sheet of thin rubber (rubber from a condom or similar material) over the site of the fang punctures, and by vigorously sucking and kneading with the teeth remove as much venom as possible during a period of 5 minutes. The rubber sheeting will prevent sucking the venom into the mouth. Wash the wound and the rubber sheeting and repeat the sucking and kneading at frequent intervals while removing the patient to the nearest medical officer or other physician.

3. If practicable, kill the snake and take it to the physician for inspection.

4. Whisky or other alcoholic drinks should *not* be given.

5. If possible, keep the patient from exerting himself, for this will increase blood flow and thus cause more venom to be absorbed.

10. Venereal diseases.—*a.* Throughout Northern Africa and Western Asia venereal diseases are prevalent. In some areas, up to 90 percent of the native populations may be infected with one or more of these diseases, which include—

(1) Syphilis.

(2) Gonorrhea.

(3) Chancroid or soft chancre.

(4) Lymphogranuloma venereum (tropical bubo).

(5) Granuloma inguinale.

b. Briefly, it may be said that in the vast majority of cases venereal disease is contracted through sexual contact, although syphilis may be acquired by kissing.

11. Sunburn; sunstroke; heat exhaustion.—*a.* Personnel accustomed to climatic conditions in the United States fail to evaluate the intensity of the sun's rays nearer the equator or in desert or arid regions. As a consequence, serious skin burns and sunstroke may occur after relatively short exposure. Persons in small boats on tropical waters may acquire severe sunburn due to reflection of the sun from the water, even though a boat with overhead protection is used. Glare from water or sand in intense sunlight often results in severe eye irritation (actinic conjunctivitis), and mechanical irritation may be produced by wind and blowing sand and dust. Exertion under hot desert conditions, with consequent fluid and salt depletion by perspiration, may cause early heat exhaustion even in physically fit individuals. See paragraph 3.

b. Precautions.—In addition to those set forth in paragraph 3, the following precautions are suggested:

(1) Wear suitable headgear (sun helmet) when exposed to the sun.

(2) Do not expose large areas of the body surface to direct rays of the sun for more than a few minutes at a time unless a thorough tan has been acquired, and then only during the early morning or the late afternoon.

(3) The use of a superior grade of dark sun glasses is advisable. The Calabar lenses now widely used by Army Air Forces personnel are satisfactory.

(4) Early recognition of the warning signs of heat stroke and heat exhaustion (dizziness, headache, blurring of vision, nausea and/or vomiting) and early first-aid treatment of these conditions. Medical attention should be obtained as soon as possible.

(5) Avoid or reduce to a minimum the consumption of alcohol.

12. Minor wounds.—Wounds do not heal rapidly in tropical climates, and infection is likely to take place. Minor wounds (cuts, scratches, abrasions, insect bites, etc.) should be treated by application of iodine or other antiseptic. Burns should be covered with boric acid ointment or sulfanilamide powder, and a dry dressing applied. All wounds should receive medical attention as soon as practicable. See FM 21–11.

13. Vaccinations.—*a.* Immunity against certain diseases may follow an attack of disease, or may be developed artificially by vaccination. *It is not to be assumed, however, that absolute protection is thus produced, or that strict observance of personal hygiene and sanitation thereby becomes any the less important.*

b. Paragraph 14 summarizes the present War Department policy on vaccinations. In addition to furnishing certain data on doses and the time required to complete vaccinations, it indicates in a general way the vaccination requirements for service in different geographical areas.

14. Summary of immunizations.—*a. General.*

(1) Due to constantly changing situations, there may be changes in the immunization program from time to

time; hence, this summary should not be considered to be an outline of permanent policy.

(2) *References.*—Section III, AR 40–210, and SGO Circular Letter No. 162, subject, Immunization, November 28, 1942.

	No. doses (basic series)	Time required (days) (basic series)
b. *Routine immunizations:*		
(1) Smallpox	1	
(2) Typhoid-paratyphoid	3	14
(3) Tetanus	3	42
c. *Special immunizations:*		
(1) Yellow fever	1	
(2) Cholera	2	7
(3) Typhus	3	14
(4) Plague	2	7

d. Immunizations required for foreign duty.

(1) *Smallpox and typhoid-paratyphoid.*—Personnel must have been vaccinated against smallpox, typhoid fever, and the paratyphoid fevers within 12 months prior to departure for foreign duty.

(2) *Tetanus.*—Initial tetanus immunization (three doses) is required. An additional dose (1 cc) is required unless the routine initial immunization or a stimulating dose has been administered within 6 months prior to departure.

(3) *Yellow fever.*—Yellow fever vaccination is required for personnel proceeding to or through certain areas (in the Eastern Hemisphere, the portion of Africa lying between latitudes 16° N. and 12° S., including the islands immediately adjacent; in the Western Hemisphere, the mainland of South America lying between latitudes 13° N. and 30° S., including the islands immediately adjacent; and the Republic of Panama, including the Canal Zone). If travel is by air, this vaccination should be done at least 2 weeks before departure in order to avoid delays en route which otherwise might arise from the quarantine requirements of certain foreign governments. Documentary proof of such vaccination is required of personnel traveling by air, particularly in India and certain other British-controlled countries. (Special references: Immediate action letter from The Adjutant General (A. G. 720.3 (6–22–42), MB–SPGA–PS–M), June 29, 1942, subject, Vaccination of troops against yellow fever, and SGO

letter (SPMCE), subject, Vaccination against yellow fever, November 17, 1942.) This vaccination will ordinarily be done at the port of embarkation or staging area.

(4) *Cholera.*—Vaccination against cholera is required for personnel proceeding to or through Asia, including the Middle East and islands of the East Indies. This vaccination will ordinarily be done at the port of embarkation or staging area.

(5) *Typhus.*—Typhus vaccination is required for personnel proceeding to or through Asia, Africa, Europe (including the British Isles), and the mountainous regions of Central and South America (including Mexico but excepting Panama). This vaccination will ordinarily be done at the port of embarkation or staging area.

(6) *Plague.*—Plague vaccine is to be administered only when personnel are under serious threat of exposure to epidemics of human plague. There is no indication at this time for the administration of plague vaccine to personnel before departure from the United States.

e. Records.—The responsibility for the completion and forwarding of permanent immunization records of enlisted personnel lies directly with the organization commanders. In order to insure the proper immunization status of personnel in his command, and to prevent unnecessary delay and undesirable repetition of the various procedures, each commander should devote particular attention to the fulfillment of this duty. See paragraph 5, AR 345–125; section III, AR 40–210; and paragraph 5*b* and *d*, AR 615–250.

[A. G. 720 (3–28–43).]

BY ORDER OF THE SECRETARY OF WAR:

G. C. MARSHALL,
Chief of Staff.

OFFICIAL:

J. A. ULIO,
Major General,
The Adjutant General.

O

Lightning Source UK Ltd.
Milton Keynes UK
UKHW041526250219
337978UK00014B/2036/P